# The Lastest Copycat Cookbook

Fantastic and ea       ;
restaurants for beginners.
The latest recipes from Red Lobster,
Panera, Olive Garden and all the others.

**Marina Grant**

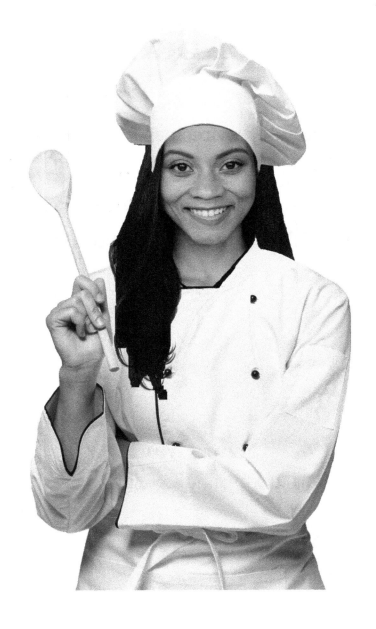

# TABLE OF CONTENTS

TABLE OF CONTENTS..........................................................................3

INTRODUCTION .................................................................................5

BREAKFAST AND BRUNCH RECIPES ...........................................10
   CHICKEN FAJITAS................................................................... 10
   MUSHROOM JACK CHICKEN FAJITAS ................................. 13
   GAME DAY CHILI.................................................................... 17
   ROASTED TURKEY, APPLE AND CHEDDAR ...................... 19
   TUNA SALAD SANDWICH ..................................................... 21
   LENTIL QUINOA BOWL WITH CHICKEN ........................... 22
   PANERA'S MAC & CHEESE.................................................... 24

PASTA RECIPES.............................................................................26
   MACARONI AND CHEESE...................................................... 26
   PEA PESTO PAPPARDELLE .................................................. 28
   BUCATINI WITH WINTER PESTO AND SWEET POTATOES ....... 29
   BEEF STROGANOFF ............................................................... 31
   TURKEY MEATBALLS OVER ZUCCHINI NOODLES ............. 33

MAIN RECIPES..............................................................................35
   LOBSTER TAILS...................................................................... 35
   TOFU & BOK CHOY SALAD .................................................. 37
   SHRIMP SCAMPI & CAPRESE TOMATOES .......................... 40
   CREAMY MUSHROOM PORK CHOPS ................................... 43
   CREAMY TUSCAN CHICKEN ................................................ 46
   GREEK SALMON ................................................................... 48
   STEAK BITES & CHIMICHURRI SAUCE .............................. 50
   LOBSTER BISQUE................................................................... 53
   SEARED SCALLOP RISOTTO ................................................ 54
   BOURSIN CHEESE STUFFED CHICKEN ............................... 56
   KETO-FRIED CHICKEN .......................................................... 59
   CAULIFLOWER SUSHI ........................................................... 61
   CHEESY BURRITO SKILLET.................................................. 63
   CHEESE TACO SHELLS........................................................... 65
   PORK RIND TORTILLAS ........................................................ 67
   MUSHROOM MASALA............................................................ 69

BEEF AND EGGPLANT KEBAB ........................................................... 71
SIX-INGREDIENT PIZZA .................................................................. 73

## APPETIZER RECIPES ...................................................................75

PANDA EXPRESS® CHICKEN POT STICKERS ...................................... 75
PANDA EXPRESS® CREAM CHEESE RANGOON ................................... 76
PANDA EXPRESS® CHICKEN EGG ROLL .......................................... 77
PANDA EXPRESS® VEGGIE SPRING ROLL......................................... 80
PF CHANG® HOT AND SOUR SOUP.................................................. 83
PF CHANG® LETTUCE WRAPS ....................................................... 85
PF CHANG® SHRIMP DUMPLINGS.................................................. 87

## DESSERT RECIPES ......................................................................89

MAPLE BUTTER BLONDIE ............................................................. 89
APPLE CHIMI CHEESECAKE .......................................................... 91
TRIPLE CHOCOLATE MELTDOWN .................................................. 93
CHOCOLATE MOUSSE DESSERT SHOOTER........................................ 96
DEADLY CHOCOLATE SIN.............................................................. 98
ORANGE CREAMSICLE CAKE ....................................................... 100
CINNAMON APPLE TURNOVER...................................................... 102
BURGER KING'S HERSHEY'S SUNDAE PIE ...................................... 104

## MEXICAN RECIPES ....................................................................106

FAJITA BURGERS....................................................................... 106
SPICY MEXICAN QUINOA ........................................................... 109
SOUTH OF THE BORDER PESTO.................................................... 111
EL POLLO SOUP....................................................................... 112
RESTAURANT-STYLE LATIN RICE ................................................ 114
CANELA BROWNIES................................................................... 116

## CONCLUSION ...........................................................................118

# INTRODUCTION

Meals in the restaurant can contain several unhealthy ingredients. There is also much more than what you lack when you feed on a take-outs.

These are some explanations of why you should consider having your cooking dinner tonight!

A Nutrient-Dense Plate

If prepared food arrives from outside the home, you typically have limited knowledge about salt, sugar, and processed oils. For a fact, we also apply more to our meal when it is served to the table. You will say how much salt, sugar, and oil are being used to prepare meals at home.

Increased Fruit and Vegetable Intake

The typical western diet loses both the weight and durability of plant foods we need to preserve. Many People eat only two fresh fruit and vegetables a day, while at least five portions are required. Tons of premade food, like restaurant food goods, restrict fruit and vegetable parts.

By supplying you with the convenience of cooking at home, you have complete control over your food. The message to note is that your attention will continue with the intake of more fruit and vegetables. Attach them to your cooking, snack them, or exchange them with your relatives on their way. Then take steps towards organic alternatives. It is always better to eat entire fruits and vegetables, whether or not organic, than processed foods.

Save Money and Use What You Have

Just because you haven't visited your local health food or food store this week doesn't mean you get stuck with taking in. Open your cupboard and fridge and see what you can make for a meal. It can be as easy as gluten-free rice, roasted tomatoes, carrots, frozen vegetables, and lemon juice. This simple meal is packed with fiber, protein, vitamins, and minerals. Best of all, in less than 30 minutes, it is delicious and can be prepared. You can save up your money in the long run and allows you sufficient food to share with or break the next day.

Sensible Snacking

Bringing premade snacks saves time, but everything goes back to what's in these products still. Don't worry, you can still have your guilty pleasures, but there is a way to make them more nutritious and often taste better. Swap your chips and dip the chopped vegetables into hummus. Create your snacks with bagged potato chips or carrots. Take a bowl and make your popcorn on top of your stove or in the popcorn machine. You can manage the amount of salt, sugar, and oil added.

Share Your Delicious Health

Once you make your recipes, you are so proud of your achievements. Furthermore, the food tastes amazing. Don't confuse me now—some of your inventive recipes won't taste the same thing, but friends and family will love your cuisine with constant practice and experimentation. You will see them enjoy the best nutritious food because of you and your faith in spreading health and love.

It Gives You a Chance to Reconnect

Having that chance to cook together helps you reconnect with your partner and your loved ones. Cooking also has other benefits. The American Psychological Association says that working together with new things—like learning a new recipe—can help maintain a relationship.

It's Proven to Be Healthier

Many researchers say that those who eat more often than not have a healthier diet overall. Such studies also show that in restaurants, menus, salt, saturated fat, total fat, and average calories are typically higher than in-house diets.

You have complete control over your food, whether you put fresh products together or shipped them straight to your door using a company like Plated. It can make a difference in your overall health.

It's Easier to Watch Your Calories

The average fast-food order is between 1,100 and 1,200 calories in total—nearly all the highly recommended daily calorie intake is 1,600 to 2,400 calories by a woman and almost two thirds (2,000 to 3,000 calories) a man daily. So, think again if you felt the independent restaurants so smaller chains would do well. Such products suck up an average of 1.327 calories per meal of additional calories.

Creating your food ensures you can guarantee that the portion sizes and calories are where you want them. Recipes also come with nutritional information and tips for sizing, which ease this.

It's a Time Saver

Part of shopping is to wait for food to come or travel to get it. It may take much more time, depending on where you live, what time you order, and whether or not the delivery person is good at directions!

It doesn't have to take much time to cook at home if you don't want it. You remove the need to search for ingredients or foodstuffs by using a service like Plated. Everything you need is at your house, in the exact amount that you use.

It's Personalized

Cooking at home gives you the chance to enjoy the food you want, how you like it. For starters, with Plated, if you want your meat more well-done or less sweet, the formula includes suggested changes.

Enjoying the Process

Once you come back home from a busy day, there is little more enjoyable than disconnecting from work emails, voicemails, unfinished assignments, or homework. Cooking at home presents you with a break from your routine and space for imagination. Rather than listen to noisy messages, you should put on the radio, collect spices, and reflect on the sizzle's odors on the stove or roast vegetables. It may stun you on how much you might like it when you make a daily habit of preparing food.

If your breakfast is great, lunch soup, or fresh tomato sauce for dinner, home cooking is a worthy investment. In return for your time and energy in preparation, you will benefit richly— from cost savings to fun with friends.

And the more you enjoy cooking in the kitchen, the more you get to make fantastic food!

# BREAKFAST AND BRUNCH RECIPES

## Chicken Fajitas

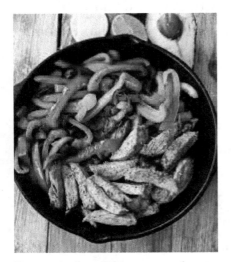

Preparation Time: 15 minutes

Cooking Time: 30 minutes

Servings: 6

**Ingredients**

For Vegetable Finishing Sauce:

- 2 tablespoon water
- ½ teaspoon lime juice, fresh
- 5 boneless skinless chicken breasts
- 2 large white onions sliced into ½" strips
- 3 bell peppers sliced into ½" strips

- Flour tortillas
- 2 teaspoon soy sauce
- ¼ teaspoon black pepper
- 2 tablespoon olive oil
- ¼ teaspoon salt

For Chicken Marinade:

- 1/3 cup lime juice, freshly squeezed
- 1 teaspoon garlic, minced
- ½ teaspoon liquid smoke
- 1 tablespoon white vinegar
- ½ teaspoon chili powder
- 1 tablespoon soy sauce
- ½ teaspoon cayenne pepper
- 2 tablespoon vegetable oil
- ¼ teaspoon onion powder
- 1 teaspoon salt
- 1/3 cup water
- ¼ teaspoon black pepper

For Toppings, Optional:

- Grated cheddar cheese, salsa, guacamole, sour cream, Pico de Gallo, shredded lettuce

**Directions**

1. Combine the entire Chicken Marinade ingredients together in a small bowl; whisk well until completely combined. Pierce each chicken breast in several places using a large fork & then place the chicken breasts in a glass baking dish, medium-sized. Add the Chicken

Marinade to the baking dish; cover & let refrigerate for overnight.

2. Over medium-high heat in a large cast iron skillet; heat the olive oil until hot & sauté the peppers for 5 to 7 minutes then add the onions. Continue to sauté until onions & peppers turn soft, for 15 to 20 minutes more, stirring every now and then.

3. In the meantime, place a separate fry pan or skillet over medium-high heat. Place the marinated chicken breasts into the hot pan & cook for 15 to 20 minutes, until done, flipping after every 10 minutes.

4. Whisk the entire Vegetable Finishing Sauce ingredients together in a small bowl. When the onions and peppers are done; decrease the heat to medium low and add in the Vegetable Finishing Sauce; let simmer for a couple of more minutes.

5. Once chicken breasts are cooked through, transfer them to a clean, large cutting board & slice it thinly. Place the onions, peppers and chicken on a flour tortilla. Top with the optional topping ingredients, as desired. Serve immediately & enjoy.

**Nutrition:** 891 calories 62.3g total fats 41.3g protein

# Mushroom Jack Chicken Fajitas

Preparation Time: 10 minutes

Cooking Time: 45 minutes

Servings: 4

**Ingredients**

For Chipotle Garlic Butter:

- 8 garlic cloves, finely minced
- ¼ cup canned chipotle peppers
- 1 teaspoon each of ground black pepper & salt
- 1/3 cup unsalted butter, softened

For Caramelized Onions:

- 1 ½ tablespoons white sugar
- 6 medium yellow or white onions; sliced into ¼ to ½" thick slices; separating them into rings
- 1 ½ tablespoons balsamic vinegar
- ¼ cup vegetable stock
- 1 ½ tablespoons butter, unsalted
- ½ teaspoon salt
- 1 ½ tablespoons vegetable oil

For Fajitas:

- 2 pounds chicken breast, boneless and skinless
- 1 tablespoon chipotle powder
- 2 tablespoons Cajun seasoning
- 1 teaspoon ground black pepper
- 2 cups green peppers
- 1/3 cup fresh cilantro, minced
- 2 tablespoons vegetable oil

- 1 cup Monterey Jack cheese, shredded
- 2 cups cremini mushrooms, sliced
- ½ cup green onion, minced
- Ground black pepper & salt to taste
- 2 tablespoons lime juice, freshly squeezed
- 1 ½ teaspoons salt

To Serve:

- ½ cup sour cream
- 12 corn or flour tortillas
- ¼ cup canned jalapeños, sliced
- 1 cup Monterey Jack cheese, shredded
- ¼ cup guacamole

## Directions

Caramelize the Onions:

1. Over moderate heat in a shallow pan; heat the butter until melted. Scatter the sliced onions on top of the melted butter and then drizzle with the oil; slowly cook for 9 minutes

2. Decrease the heat to medium-low; give the onions a good stir and add the vinegar and sugar; toss & stir until mixed well.

3. Stir in the broth. To prevent the onions from burning; don't forget to scrape up any caramelized bits from the bottom of your pan & stir every now and then.

4. Once the onions are browned well & very soft, after 10 to 15 minutes more of cooking; remove them from the heat.

Preparing the Butter:

1. Now, over medium heat in a small saucepan, heat 2 tablespoons of the butter until melted and then add the minced garlic; cook for 8 to 10 minutes, until the garlic turns fragrant and begins to brown.

2. Remove the butter from heat and place in the fridge until chilled, for 15 minutes. In a small bowl; combine the garlic butter together with softened butter, chipotle & salt.

3. Mesh all of the ingredients together with a fork. Season the mixture with more of salt & ground black pepper, if required. Using a plastic wrap; cover the seasoned butter & store it in the fridge until ready to use.

For the Fajitas:

1. Slice the chicken breast into ½" strips; rubbing them with the chipotle powder, Cajun seasoning, lime juice, pepper and salt. Let rest while you heat the pan.

2. Now, over high heat in a cast iron pan; heat half of the oil, stir in half of the chicken strips; cook until cooked through & well-browned. Transfer the cooked chicken to a plate & cook the leftover chicken strips.

3. Add the sliced mushrooms to the hot pan; ensure that you don't add more of oil or rinse the mushrooms. Bring the heat to medium-high & cook until the mushrooms turn brown & begin to crisp, undisturbed. Sprinkle them with a very small quantity of salt.

4. Carefully flip the mushrooms & continue to cook for 5 to 7 more minutes, until both sides turn browned & they are completely cooked. Transfer them to the plate with the cooked chicken.

5. Add the leftover oil to the hot pan. When it starts to shimmer and starts to smoke, add in the green peppers & lightly sprinkle them with a very small amount of salt, stirring occasionally.

6. When the peppers begin to soften, push them so that they sit around the edge of the pan; decrease the heat to low.

7. Add the caramelized onions to the middle of your pan, pushing them so that the peppers and onions cover any exposed portions of the pan.

8. Place the cooked chicken strips over the onions. Dot the onions, peppers and chicken with the chipotle butter sauce.

9. Sprinkle the chicken with the shredded cheese. Layer the cooked mushrooms on top of the cheese & dot the mushrooms with ½ to 1 tablespoon more of butter.

10. Close and sit for 5 minutes, on low heat. Once the chicken is warmed through & the cheese is completely melted, scatter the cilantro and green onions on top.

11. Serve the fajitas immediately, in the cast iron pan. Warm the tortillas & serve the salsa, jalapeños, sour cream, guacamole and extra cheese on the side

**Nutrition:** 894 calories 60.9g total fats 40.9g protein

# Game Day Chili

Preparation Time: 25 minutes

Cooking Time: 3 hours and 5 minutes

Servings: 13

**Ingredients**

- 1 can tomato paste (6-ounce)
- 2 pounds ground chuck
- 1 onion, medium, chopped
- 3 cans tomato sauce (8-ounce)
- 1 can beef broth (14 ½ ounce)
- 2 cans pinto beans, rinsed & drained (15-ounce)
- 1 can chopped green chilis (4.5-ounce)
- 3 - 4 garlic cloves, minced
- 1 bottle dark beer (12-ounce)
- 2 tablespoons chili powder
- 1 tablespoon Worcestershire sauce
- 2 teaspoons ground cumin
- 1 teaspoon paprika
- 1 to 2 teaspoons ground red pepper
- Pickled jalapeño pepper slices, for garnish
- 1 teaspoon hot sauce

**Directions**

1. Cook ground chuck together with chopped onion and minced garlic cloves over medium heat in a Dutch oven, stirring frequently until the meat crumbles & is no longer pink from inside; drain well.

2. Combine the meat mixture with beans & the leftover ingredients (except the one for garnish) in the Dutch oven; bring everything together to a boil. Decrease the heat & let simmer until thickened, for 3 hours. Garnish the recipe with pickled jalapeno pepper slices.

**Nutrition:** 884 calories 58g total fats 40g protein

# Roasted Turkey, Apple and Cheddar

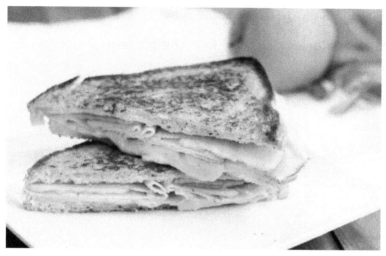

Preparation Time: 5 minutes

Cooking Time: 5 minutes

Servings: 4

## Ingredients

- 8-10 ounces thick sliced roasted turkey breast
- 3 tablespoons Dijon mustard
- 1 gala apple thinly sliced
- ½ red onion, sliced thinly
- 4 ounces sharp white cheddar cheese sliced
- 8 slices Cranberry Walnut bread
- 1 tablespoon honey
- 8 pieces of lettuce about size of bread

## Directions

1. Mix honey together with mustard and prepare the Honey mustard. Spread this mixture over the bread slices.

---

2. Layer 4 slices of the bread with lettuce, turkey, cheese, apple and onion. Place the leftover slices of bread over the sandwiches; slice & serve.

**Nutrition:** 817 calories 54g total fats 38g protein

# Tuna Salad Sandwich

Preparation Time: 10 minutes

Cooking Time: 10 minutes

Servings: 3

## Ingredients

- 1 can tuna, drained (6 ounce)
- 1 teaspoon Dijon-style prepared mustard
- ¼ teaspoon ground black pepper
- 1 teaspoon sweet pickle relish
- 1 teaspoon mayonnaise
- ¼ cup chopped onion
- 1 celery stalk, chopped

## Directions

1. Mash the tuna using a fork in a small bowl. Add pickle relish together with mayonnaise, celery, mustard, onion & black pepper; give everything a good stir until evenly combined. Let chill; serve & enjoy.

**Nutrition:** 801 calories 51g total fats 36g protein

# Lentil Quinoa Bowl with Chicken

Preparation Time: 5 minutes
Cooking Time: 15 minutes
Servings: 2

## Ingredients

- 8 ounces cooked chicken or 2 boiled eggs
- 1 cup cooked lentils
- ½ tablespoon oil
- 1 garlic clove, minced
- ¼ teaspoon paprika
- 3 cups chicken broth
- ½ onion, chopped
- 1 cup fresh spinach
- ¼ cup sun-dried tomatoes
- 1 cup chopped kale
- ¼ cup uncooked quinoa
- 1 bay leaf
- A dash of cayenne
- ½ tbsp. Miso Paste dissolved in 1 tbsp. water
- Pepper and salt to Taste

## Directions

1. At medium heat in a big saucepan; cook oil until hot. Add onion & garlic; sauté until onions are translucent & fragrant, for a couple of minutes.

2. Add quinoa together with bay leaf, broth, sun-dried tomatoes, lentils, Miso mixture and seasoning to the pan. Bring everything together to a boil and then decrease the heat to low. Cover & let simmer until quinoa is cooked through, for 10 to 15 minutes.

3. Mix in spinach and kale; let them gently wilt in the mixture. Transfer the mixture into 2 separate bowls; top each bowl with 4 ounces of chicken or a sliced egg.

**Nutrition:** 863 calories 52g total fats 33g protein

# Panera's Mac & Cheese

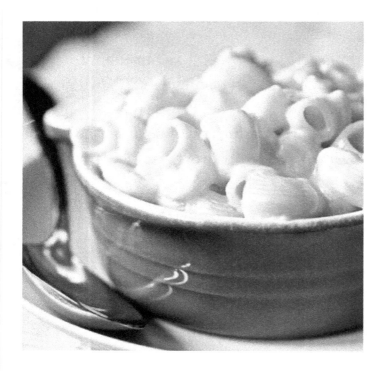

Preparation Time: 10 minutes

Cooking Time: 15 minutes

Servings: 2

## Ingredients

- 1 package rigatoni pasta (16-ounce)
- ½ teaspoon Dijon mustard
- 6 Slices white American cheese, sliced into thin strips
- ¼ cup all-purpose flour
- 8 ounces extra-sharp white Vermont cheddar, shredded
- ¼ teaspoon hot sauce
- 2 ½ cup milk

- ¼ cup butter
- 1 teaspoon kosher salt

## Directions

1. Prepare the pasta as per the directions mentioned on the package.
2. Now, over low heat in a large saucepan; heat the butter until completely melted. Cook flour for a minute, whisking constantly.
3. Slowly stir in the milk; adjust heat to medium and cook, whisking until mixture starts to bubble and thickens. Remove the pan from heat.
4. Add mustard, cheeses, hot sauce and salt; continue to stir until the sauce is smooth & cheese melts.
5. Stir in the pasta & cook over medium heat for a minute. Serve immediately & enjoy.

**Nutrition:** 846 calories 55g total fats 37g protein

# PASTA RECIPES

## Macaroni and Cheese

Preparation Time: 5 minutes

Cooking Time: 25 minutes

Servings: 4 - 6

**Ingredients:**

- 2 tablespoons butter
- 2 tablespoons flour
- 1 teaspoon salt
- 1 teaspoon dry mustard
- 2½ cups milk
- ½ pound (about 2 cups) cheddar (divided)
- ½ pound (2 cups) elbow macaroni, cooked

**Directions:**

1. Preheat the oven to 375°F.
2. Cook butter in a saucepan, then stir in the flour, salt, and mustard.
3. Whisk in the milk and stir constantly until the sauce begins to thicken.
4. Stir in 1½ cups of the cheese. Continue to stir until melted, then remove from the heat.
5. Add the cooked elbow macaroni and the cheese sauce to a buttered casserole dish. Stir until the macaroni is covered with sauce. Top with the remaining cheese and

bake for 25 minutes or until the top is browned and the cheese is bubbly.

**Nutrition:** 215 Calories 17g Fat 8g Protein

# Pea Pesto Pappardelle

Preparation Time: 10 minutes

Cooking Time: 15 minutes

Servings: 4

**Ingredients:**

- 12 oz pappardelle
- 1 1/2 c fresh peas
- 1 tsp. lemon zest
- 1/2 ricotta
- Salt
- Pepper
- Chopped chives, for serving

**Directions:**

1. Pappardelle to cook. Reserve 1/2 cup water for cooking; drain and return the pasta to the pot.
2. While cooking pasta, in the food processor, pulse 1 cup of peas to chop roughly. Add ricotta and lemon zest, and pulse to combine a few times (some chopped peas should still be present).
3. Salt and pepper to season.
4. Add a mixture of ricotta, remaining 1/2 cup peas and pasta water; toss to combine. Where desired, sprinkle with chopped chives.

**Nutrition:** 245 Calories 13g Fat 6g Protein

# Bucatini with Winter Pesto and Sweet Potatoes

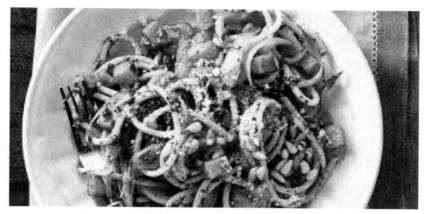

Preparation Time: 10 minutes

Cooking Time: 18 minutes

Servings: 4

## Ingredients:

- 1 large sweet potato
- 1 medium red onion
- 1/3 cups olive oil
- 4 cups torn kale
- 1/2 cup fresh flat-leaf parsley
- 2 oz. grated Parmesan cheese
- 1 clove garlic
- 2 tsp. lemon zest
- 12 oz. bucatini

## Directions:

1. Prep oven to 425F. On a rimmed baking sheet, toss potato, onion and 2 tablespoons of oil together.
2. Season with pepper and salt. Bake, stirring once, for 24 to 26 minutes until potato and onion are tender.
3. In the meantime, put the kale and parsley in a food processor. Pulse four to five times, until chopped.
4. Add parmesan, lemon zest, garlic and juice.
5. Pulse, scrape down the sides as needed, 10 to 12 times until finely chopped.
6. With the machine running, add over the feed tube slowly the remaining 1/3 cup oil. Season with pepper and salt.
7. Cook pasta following to the instructions of the package, and reserve 1/4 cup of pasta water before draining.
8. Toss plates of pasta with roasted vegetables, pesto, and water for pasta.
9. Serve topped with pine and Parmesan nuts.

**Nutrition:** 243 Calories 17g Fat 10g Protein

# Beef Stroganoff

Preparation Time: 5 minutes

Cooking Time: 25 minutes

Servings: 4

**Ingredients:**

- 2 tbsp. olive oil
- 10 oz. cremini mushrooms (sliced)
- Kosher salt
- Pepper
- 1 lb. lean beef sirloin (thinly sliced)
- 2 cloves garlic (finely chopped)
- 2 tbsp. Dijon mustard
- 1/2 c. dry white wine
- 3 1/2 low-sodium beef broth
- 8 oz. fusilli pasta
- 3 tbsp. crème fraiche or sour cream

**Directions:**

1. Steam on medium-high 1 tablespoon of olive oil in a large skillet.
2. Add the cremini mushrooms, season with salt and pepper and cook for 5 minutes, stirring occasionally until browned. Move to the pot.
3. Return pan to medium heat, add 1 spoonful of olive oil, season thinly sliced lean beef sirloin with salt and pepper, and cook well.

---

4. Attach the garlic and cook for 1 minute, then mix in the mustard for Dijon.
5. Add and cook dry white wine, scrape any brown pieces, then add low-sodium beef broth and bring to a simmer.
6. Add the fusilli pasta and mushrooms with their juices and simmer until pasta is al dente, stirring regularly, 14 to 18 minutes.
7. Stir in crème fraiche or sour cream, and add salt and pepper to season.

**Nutrition:** 268 Calories 13g Fat 8g Protein

# Turkey Meatballs Over Zucchini Noodles

Preparation Time: 5 minutes

Cooking Time: 15 minutes

Servings: 4

## Ingredient:

- 1 lb. ground turkey
- 1/4 cup seasoned dry breadcrumbs
- 1 pc. egg
- 3 tbsp. fresh flat-leaf parsley
- 1 1/2 oz. Parmesan cheese
- 2 garlic cloves
- 2 tbsp. extra-virgin olive oil
- 1 (25-oz.) jar marinara sauce
- 4 medium zucchinis
- 4 oz. Provolone cheese

## Directions:

1. Combine each salt and pepper in a bowl with turkey, breadcrumbs, egg, parmesan, 1 garlic clove, and 1/2 teaspoon.
2. Form into meatballs of 12 (1 ½" to 2"). Heat 1 tablespoon of oil over medium heat in a large skillet.
3. Attach the meatballs and cook for 4 to 6 minutes, turning occasionally, until brown on all sides.

4. Reduce heat in marinara to medium-low, and stir gently. Simmer until meatballs are cooked through and the sauce thickened, turning meatballs periodically, 14 to 16 minutes.
5. Meanwhile, over medium to high heat, heat remaining tablespoon oil in a medium skillet.
6. Add the zucchini and remaining garlic, and cook for 2 to 3 minutes until tender and moist. Salt and pepper to season.
7. In top spot, heat broiler to high with rack. Sprinkle over meatballs with provolone. Broil for 4 minutes. Serve the meatballs over Parmesan-toped noodles.

**Nutrition:** 246 Calories 17g Fat 9g Protein

# MAIN RECIPES

## Lobster Tails

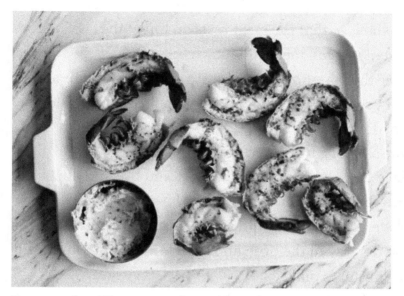

Preparation Time: 10 minutes

Cooking Time: 10 minutes

Servings: 1

**Ingredients:**

- 1 lobster tail (per person)
- 1/8 cup butter per lobster
- ½ garlic clove, finely chopped
- ½ tsp of paprika
- salt & pepper to taste
- ½ scallion, finely chopped
- 1 lemon wedge for serving

**Directions:**

1. Preheat the oven to 450°F and set the oven to broil.
2. Cut through the lobster shell, from top to tail, using a sharp set of shears. Leave the tail intact so the shell doesn't completely open up.
3. Using a fork, lift the meat out of the shell and then close the shell, so that the meat rests on top of the shell. Keep the tail and tail meat still intact.
4. Place the butter in a small bowl and microwave for about 10-15 seconds until the butter is melted. Set it aside to cool down.
5. Line a baking tray with foil.
6. Place the lobster on a baking tray and brush the lobster with the melted butter, sprinkle the garlic clove over the lobster, then season with salt, pepper and paprika.
7. Pop the tray in the oven and broil for 7-10 minutes until the lobster is pink.
8. Garnish with chopped scallions and serve with a slice of lemon for squeezing over the lobster.

**Nutrition:** 252 Calories 23g Fat 11g Protein

# Tofu & Bok Choy Salad

Preparation Time: 7 hours
Cooking Time: 40 minutes
Servings: 3

**Ingredients:**

For the Tofu:

- 15 oz of firm tofu
- 1 tbsp of soy sauce
- 1 tbsp of sesame oil
- 2 tsps. of garlic paste
- 1 tbsp of rice wine vinegar
- ½ a lemon's worth of juice
- ¼ tsp paprika
- ¼ tsp black pepper
- 1 tbsp of water

For the Bok Choy Salad:

- 9 oz of bok choy, chopped
- 1 scallion, chopped
- 2 tbsps. of chopped cilantro
- 3 tbsps. of coconut oil
- 1 tbsp of coconut shavings
- 2 tbsps. of soy sauce
- 1 tbsp of sambal oelek (this can be substituted for another hot sauce)
- 1 tbsp of unsalted peanut butter
- ½ lime's worth of juice

- 7 drops of liquid stevia
- ¼ tbsp of sesame seeds
- ¼ tsp of chili flakes

**Directions:**

1. Prepare the tofu by wrapping the tofu in a kitchen towel and placing a weighted object on top of it (such as a skillet). Leave the tofu to press for 4-6 hours, until the tofu has dried out. Check on the towel to see if it needs to be swapped for a dry one halfway through the drying process.

2. Once the tofu has dried, prepare the marinade sauce: in a small bowl, mix in the soy sauce, sesame oil, garlic paste, vinegar, lemon juice, water, paprika and black pepper. Stir well to combine.

3. Cut the tofu into squares of about 2" each and place the squares in a plastic bag. Add the marinade into the bag and set it aside to marinate for 30 minutes (you can leave it to marinate for longer/overnight if desired).

4. Once the tofu has properly marinated, preheat the oven to 350°F and line a baking tray with parchment paper. Place the tofu onto the tray and bake for 30-35 minutes until the tofu is lightly browned.

5. While the tofu bakes, prepare the salad dressing: add the scallion, cilantro, coconut oil, coconut shavings, soy sauce, sambal oelek (or spicy sauce substitute), peanut butter, lime juice, liquid stevia, sesame seeds, and chili flakes into a small bowl and mix well to combine all of the flavors.

6. To assemble the salad, add a handful of the bok choy, a few squares of tofu and drizzle the salad dressing over. You can sprinkle a few more chili flakes on top of the salad for an extra spicy kick.

**Nutrition** 398 Calories 30g Fat 24g Protein

# Shrimp Scampi & Caprese Tomatoes

Preparation Time: 10 minutes

Cooking Time: 35 minutes

Servings: 4

**Ingredients:**

For the shrimp scampi:

- 4 tbsps. of butter, unsalted
- 3 tbsps. of olive oil
- 1 shallot, thinly sliced
- 3 tbsps. of garlic paste
- ½ cup of broth/pinot grigio (or any dry, white wine)
- 1 tbsp of lemon juice
- ¼ tsp of chili flakes
- a pinch of salt
- ¼ cup of parsley
- 1 lb. of shrimp

For the Caprese Tomatoes:

- 6 whole tomatoes
- 1 tbsp of olive oil
- 2 tbsps. of balsamic vinegar
- 1 tsp of mixed herb spice
- 6 slices of mozzarella/cheddar
- 6 basil leaves
- a handful of rockets for serving
- salt & pepper to taste

For the Dressing:

- a handful of basil
- 1 tsp of garlic, minced/paste
- 2 tbsps. of olive oil
- salt to taste

**Directions:**

1. Preheat the oven to 350°F and prepare a baking tray (a muffin tray is more preferable for this recipe, so that the tomatoes don't roll around on the tray).

2. Wash the tomatoes and halve them horizontally. Place them on the baking/muffin tray with the cut side facing upwards.

3. Drizzle the olive oil and balsamic vinegar, then season generously with the herb spice, salt, and pepper.

4. Add a slice of mozzarella/cheddar and basil to the 3 bottom halves of the tomatoes, then place the top halves of the tomatoes back on the bottom halves (creating a tomato sandwich).

5. Place the tomatoes in the oven for 20-25 minutes, until the tomatoes' skin starts to blister and the cheese has melted.

6. While the tomatoes are roasting, prepare the shrimp: place a medium saucepan over medium heat and add in the butter, olive oil, shallot and garlic to the pan. Stir the mixture for about 3 minutes until the butter has melted and the shallot has softened.

7. Pour the pinot grigio, lemon juice, chili flakes and salt into the pan and reduce the heat to medium-low. Stir the

seasoning into the mix for about 3 minutes until fragrant and the mixture is reduced to half.

8. Add in the shrimp and parsley. Cook for another 5 minutes until the shrimp is pink in color. Lower the heat to the lowest temperature and cover the pan until you're ready to plate the shrimp (this is to keep it warm until ready to serve).

9. Next, make the dressing for the tomatoes: combine the basil, garlic, olive oil, salt, and pepper into a blender and blend until the ingredients are finely chopped. Set aside.

10. Once the tomatoes are ready, set them aside for 5 minutes to cool down. Add a few leaves of the rocket onto each plate, then place 2 tomatoes onto the rocket. Drizzle the tomatoes and rocket with the dressing, then add a spoonful or two of the shrimps onto each plate. Serve warm.

**Nutrition** 542 Calories 38g Fat 31g Protein

# Creamy Mushroom Pork Chops

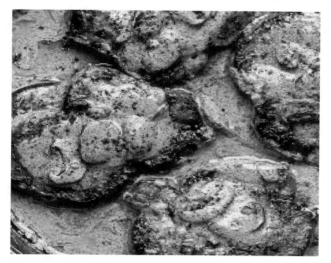

Preparation Time: 10 minutes

Cooking Time: 20 minutes

Servings: 4

**Ingredients:**

- 4 bone-in pork chops
- 2 tsps. of salt, divided
- 1 tsp of black pepper, divided
- 1 tsp of paprika
- ¼ tsp of cinnamon
- 3 tbsps. of butter
- 3 tbsp. of olive oil
- a pinch of rosemary
- 2 tsp. of thyme
- 1 tbsp of garlic paste
- ¾ cup of mushrooms (portobello preferable)

- ½ an onion, thinly sliced
- ¼ cup of broth/water
- ¾ cup of heavy cream
- 1 tsp of parsley
- a squeeze of lemon juice

**Directions:**

1. In a small bowl, combine ¾ tsp of salt, ½ tsp of black pepper, paprika and cinnamon. Mix the spices together to combine, then massage the spice into the pork chops. Make sure to evenly cover the meat. Cover the chops and set it aside.

2. Prepare a large saucepan over medium-high heat and add the butter, olive oil, rosemary and thyme into the pan, stirring the contents while the butter melts.

3. Add the chops into the pan once the butter has melted, and cook the chops for about 5 minutes on either side, until the chops have browned. Remove the chops from the pan and set it aside to cool down.

4. In the same saucepan, add the onions and garlic paste and stir it over medium heat for about 2 minutes, until the onions are fragrant and have softened.

5. Add the mushrooms into the pan and stir for another 3 minutes, until the mushrooms have browned and softened.

6. Pour the heavy cream and broth into the pan and reduce the heat to a medium-low. Slowly stir the mixture for about 3-4 minutes until it thickens, then season it with a pinch of salt and pepper.

7.  Remove from heat and drizzle the sauce over the pork chops. Garnish with some parsley and a squeeze of lemon juice. Serve warm.

**Nutrition** 477 Calories 34g Fat 36g Protein

# Creamy Tuscan Chicken

Preparation Time: 10 minutes

Cooking Time: 20 minutes

Servings: 4

**Ingredients:**

- 4 chicken breast pieces
- 1 ½ tsp of garlic paste/powder
- 1 tsp of paprika
- ½ tsp of cumin
- ¼ tsp of turmeric
- 2 tbsps. of butter
- salt to taste
- 1 cup of heavy cream
- ½ cup of oil-packed sun-dried tomatoes
- a pinch of white pepper
- 1 cup of spinach
- 2 tbsps. of parsley
- ¼ cup of crumbled feta cheese

**Directions:**

1. Place the chicken breast pieces into a large bowl and add in the garlic paste, paprika, cumin, turmeric and salt. Mix the contents together to evenly coat the chicken.

2. Place a large pan over medium heat and add the butter into the pan. Stir the butter for about 1 minute until it melts, then add the chicken breast pieces into the pan.

3. Fry the chicken for about 6-7 minutes on either side until the chicken is cooked & browned from the seasoning, then remove the chicken from the pan and set aside.

4. Pour the heavy cream and tomatoes into the pan and stir the mixture to combine well. Sprinkle a bit of white pepper into the mix and continue to stir for about 3 minutes, then add the spinach and chicken back into the pan.

5. Allow the contents to simmer for about 3-4 minutes. Sprinkle some parsley and the feta cheese over the meal, then serve hot.

**Nutrition** 485 Calories 32g Fat    42g Protein

# Greek Salmon

Preparation Time: 15 minutes

Cooking Time: 20 minutes

Servings: 4

**Ingredients:**

For the salmon:

- 12 oz of salmon (4 fillets)
- 1 lemon, thinly sliced
- 1 red onion, thinly sliced
- salt & pepper to taste
- 1/2 tsp of ginger, grated finely
- lemon wedges for serving

For the salad:

- 1/4 cup of olive oil
- 2 lemon's worth of juice
- 1 tbsp of garlic paste
- 1 tsp of oregano
- 1/2 tsp of chili flakes
- 1 cup of feta, cubed
- 1 cup of halved cherry tomatoes
- 1/4 cup of halved & pitted olives
- 1/4 cup of cucumber, diced
- 1/4 cup of red onion, diced/sliced thinly
- 2 tbsps. of dill, chopped finely
- 1 tsp of mixed herbs
- 1/2 tsp of green chili, chopped finely

**Directions:**

1.  Preheat the oven to 375°F.
2.  Combine the olive oil, lemon juice, garlic, oregano, chili flakes and oregano in a small bowl and whisk together. Place the feta cubes into the bowl and add a pinch of salt and pepper. Toss the feta cubes in the bowl to mix well, then cover the bowl and place it in the refrigerator for 10 minutes to marinate.
3.  Prepare a baking tray and evenly layer the lemon slices and onion slices on the surface of the tray, then lay the fillets of salmon on top of the bedding (with the skin of the fillets on the base). Season the fillets with salt, pepper and the ginger, then place the tray in the oven to bake for 20 minutes, until the fish is flaky and cooked.
4.  While the salmon is cooking, prepare the salad. In a medium bowl, mix the marinated feta, tomatoes, olives, cucumbers, red onion, dill, mixed herbs and green chili in a bowl. Mix well to combine the ingredients.
5.  Place the fish fillets and top with spoonful of salad. Serve with a lemon wedge and enjoy.

**Nutrition** 358 Calories 27g Fat 23g Protein

# Steak Bites & Chimichurri Sauce

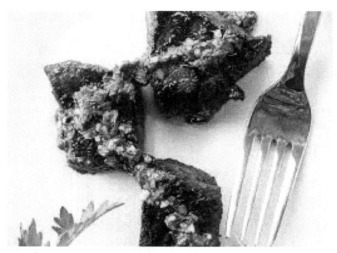

Preparation Time: 10 minutes

Cooking Time: 10 minutes

Servings: 4

**Ingredients:**

- 3 tbsps. olive oil
- 1 tbsp balsamic vinegar
- ½ of garlic paste
- 1 lb. of beef sirloin (chopped into 1 ½" chunks)
- salt & pepper for seasoning
- 1 tsp of rosemary
- 1 tbsp of oil for cooking
- salad of choice as a side option when serving

For the chimichurri sauce:

- ½ cup olive oil
- 2 tbsps. white wine vinegar
- ¾ cup of parsley, finely chopped

- 2 tbsps. of finely chopped garlic
- 2 tsps. of oregano
- ½ tsp of chili flakes
- 1 tsp of chopped chili
- a pinch of salt to taste

**Directions:**

1. Combine the olive oil, balsamic vinegar, rosemary, garlic paste, salt, and pepper in a bowl and whisk until well combined.

2. Place the steaks in a large bowl and coat them with the marinade. Mix the contents together to ensure that the meat is fully coated, then cover the bowl and set it aside to marinate for about 30 minutes.

3. While the steak is marinating, prepare the chimichurri sauce by adding all of the contents into a glass jar/enclosed bottle and shaking the mixture until well combined. Taste to check for seasoning and add more salt/chili if desired. Set the sauce aside.

4. When the steaks have marinated for long enough, place a large saucepan over medium-high heat and allow the pan to heat up for 2-5 minutes. You can test the heat by placing your hand a few inches above the pan and feel the heat.

5. Drizzle a little oil into the pan to lightly coat the surface, then add the steak bits into the pan. Allow the meat to fry for about 30-40 seconds until the bottom has browned, then flip the bits over to fry for another 30-40 seconds until the other side has browned.

6. Serve with the chimichurri sauce as a dip, and a salad of choice as a side.

**Nutrition** 356 Calories 27g Fat 24g Protein

# Lobster Bisque

Preparation Time: 20 minutes
Cooking Time: 81 minutes
Servings: 4

**Ingredients:**

- ½ red onion, chopped finely
- 2 tbsps. of garlic paste
- 1 tbsp of salt
- 1 tsp of paprika
- 1 tsp of thyme seasoning
- 3 bay leaves
- 1-star anise
- 1 tsp of peppercorn
- 2 cups of white wine
- 2 carrots, sliced thinly
- 4 celery stalks, thinly sliced
- ½ cup of tomato paste
- 1 quart of broth/water
- 1 oz of brandy
- 1 cup of heavy cream
- 24 oz of lobster chunks
- 1 tbsp of butter
- 1 tbsp of lemon juice
- parsley and chives, finely chopped, for garnish

**Directions:**

1. Combine the garlic, onion, salt, paprika, bay leaves, star anise, peppercorn and thyme into a medium pot on medium-high heat. Stir for about 1 minute until fragrant.

2. Pour in the white wine and add the carrots and celery into the mixture. Stir for about 3 minutes until the carrots have softened.

3. Add in the broth, tomato paste and brandy. Lower the heat to a medium-low, cover the pot and allow the contents to simmer for 1 hour.

4. After an hour, remove the bay leaves and star anise and discard them. Pour in the cream into the pot and bring to a simmer for another 10 minutes, then remove from heat and allow the soup to cool down.

5. Add the soup mixture into a blender and blend until smooth, then set aside.

6. Place the lobster chunks in a saucepan with the butter, and fry over medium-high heat for about 5-8 minutes until fully cooked.

7. Spoon the soup into bowls and top with lobster bits. Drizzle some lemon juice over the top and garnish with parsley and chopped chives.

**Nutrition** 220 Calories 15g Fat 12g Protein


# Seared Scallop Risotto

Preparation Time: 10 minutes
Cooking Time: 20 minutes
Servings: 4

## Ingredients:

For the Risotto:

- 3 tbsps. of butter
- 1 tbsp of garlic paste
- 1 cup of broccoli florets, cut into chunks (about 1" pieces)
- ¼ cup of scallions, chopped finely
- 4 cups of riced cauliflower
- 1 cup of heavy whipping cream
- ¾ cup of grated parmesan cheese
- salt & pepper to taste
- 1 tbsp of olive oil
- 1 green chili, chopped finely
- ¼ cup of crumbled feta cheese for topping

For the scallops:

- 1 lb. of scallops
- 2 tbsps. of butter
- 1 tbsp of olive oil
- salt & pepper to taste
- ½ green chili, chopped finely

## Directions:

1. In a medium saucepan, add the butter, garlic, broccoli and scallops into the pan and cook over a medium heat for about 3-4 minutes, allowing the broccoli to soften.
2. Pour the cauliflower rice into the pan and continue to cook whilst slowly stirring the contents, for another 3 minutes.

3. Lastly, pour the whipping cream, parmesan cheese, and salt and pepper (to taste) into the pan and cook for another 2 minutes, while still stirring. Remove from heat and set aside.

4. To prepare the scallops, dry them with a paper towel, then add them into a small frying pan, along with the butter, 1 tbsp of olive oil, salt, pepper and ½ a green chili, over a medium heat. Cook the scallops for about 5 minutes, flipping them over halfway through.

5. Transfer the scallops into a small bowl.

6. In another small bowl, combine the 1 tbsp of olive oil and the last 1 green chili, chopped. Mix together.

7. When serving, add about ½ a cup's worth of the risotto, and then top the risotto with a few scallops. Drizzle a little chili mixture over each dish and then add a little crumbled feta on top. Serve warm.

**Nutrition** 551 Calories 47g Fat 23g Protein

# Boursin Cheese Stuffed Chicken

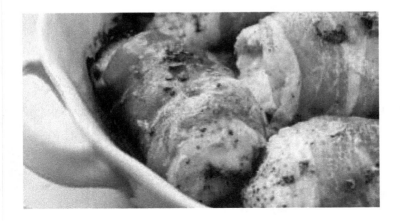

Preparation Time: 15 minutes

Cooking Time: 45 minutes

Servings: 4

**Ingredients:**

- 4 boneless chicken breast pieces
- 1 tbsp of garlic paste
- 4 oz of Boursin cheese
- ½ cup of shredded mozzarella
- 4 slices of prosciutto
- salt & pepper to taste
- ½ tsp of mixed herbs spice

**Directions:**

1. Preheat the oven to 400°F and prepare a deep-set ovenproof dish.

2. Lay the chicken breast pieces on a chopping board and pound the meat, using a meat tenderizer (alternatively, you can place plastic wrap over the meat and roll it with a rolling pin). Aim to get the breast pieces to about ¼" in thickness.

3. Season the meat with salt, pepper and garlic paste, and massage it in so that it's evenly coated and the chicken infuses the spice well while it's cooking.

4. Add a dollop of Boursin cheese on the end of each chicken breast, then sprinkle mozzarella cheese.

5. Roll the chicken breast pieces, starting from the end where the cheeses are such that you create tiny chicken rolls with cheese in the center.

6. Tightly wrap a slice of prosciutto around each chicken roll and then place the rolls into the baking dish. Sprinkle mixed herb spice over the dish.

7. Pop the baking dish in the oven and bake for 30-35 minutes until the chicken is cooked and the juices have dried up.

8. Serve warm.

**Nutrition:** 524 Calories 28g Fat 63g Protein

# Keto-Fried Chicken

Preparation Time: 10 minutes
Cooking Time: 20 minutes
Servings: 4

**Ingredients:**

- 4 chicken thigh pieces
- oil for frying
- 2 eggs
- 2 tbsps. of heavy whipping cream
- 2/3 cups of almond flour
- 2/3 cup of grated parmesan cheese
- 1 tsp of salt
- ½ tsp of black pepper
- ½ tsp of paprika
- ½ tsp of cayenne pepper

**Directions:**

1. Chop the chicken pieces into even strips and pat dry with a paper towel. Lay the chicken strips on a baking tray lined with parchment paper.
2. In a medium bowl, crack the eggs into the bowl and add in the heavy cream. Whisk the eggs and cream together until light and fluffy.
3. In another medium sized bowl, add the almond flour, parmesan cheese, salt, pepper, paprika and cayenne pepper. Stir the ingredients to combine well.
4. Coat each piece of chicken in the bowl with the dry ingredients, then dip the chicken strips into the egg-

wash bowl, and then back into the bowl with the dry ingredients.

5. Place the chicken strips back on the baking tray.

6. Place a medium pot over medium-high heat and fill the pot with 2 inches of oil. Once the oil has heated up, place the chicken strips into the oil and fry for 5 minutes, until crisp and brown. Place the fried chicken on a paper towel to drain the excess oil.

**Nutrition** 380 Calories 26g Fat 34g Protein

# Cauliflower Sushi

Preparation Time: 15 minutes

Cooking Time: 0 minutes

Servings: 4

**Ingredients:**

- 18oz of cauliflower, chopped into ½" chunks
- 3.5oz of cream cheese
- 1 spring onion, sliced thinly
- 1 tbsp of white vinegar
- 1 carrot, chopped into thin 1" strips
- ½ an avocado, cut into thin slices
- ¼ cucumber, sliced thinly
- 3.5oz of salmon/prawns/fish of your choice, cut into thin strips
- 4 seaweed sheets
- 2 tbsps. of mayonnaise, divided
- ½ tsp of paprika
- 1 tsp of sesame seeds
- salt & pepper to taste

**Directions:**

1. Add the raw cauliflower into a food processor and blend until shredded into a fine, cauliflower rice texture.
2. Pour the cream cheese, spring onion, vinegar, and a pinch of salt and pepper into the cauliflower mix. Blend the mix once more to combine the ingredients (don't

over-process the mixture, as you don't want a puree—you want to maintain the fine, grain texture).

3. Lay the seaweed wraps on a working station (the shiny side faces down). Prepare the other vegetables and fish so that it's in arm's reach when you make the sushi rolls.

4. Layer the cauliflower rice over ¾ of the seaweed sheets, leaving 2" of one of the edges free.

5. Leave 1" on the other edge, where the cauliflower rice meets the seaweed, and then horizontally layer the fish, cucumber strips, avocado strips and carrot strips.

6. Starting from the edge where the cauliflower rice meets the seaweed, start to roll the sushi together. Once you reach the other end where there's no rice, lightly dampen the seaweed with a bit of water, and stick it to the roll to close it off.

7. Cut the sushi roll in half, then again, until you have 8 equal sushi rolls from the 1 sheet of seaweed.

8. Add a dollop of mayonnaise onto each roll, then sprinkle paprika and sesame seeds on top. Enjoy the sushi with wasabi and soy sauce (or aminos).

**Nutrition** 119 Calories 8g Fat 4g Protein

# Cheesy Burrito Skillet

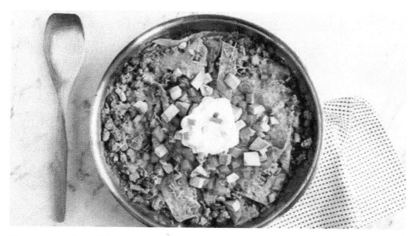

Preparation Time: 5 minutes

Cooking Time: 20 minutes

Servings: 6

**Ingredients:**

- 1 tbsp of oil
- 1 onion, diced
- 2 bell peppers, diced
- 1 tsp of mixed herb spice
- 1 lb. of ground beef
- ½ tbsp of garlic paste
- 1 can of diced tomato & chili
- ½ cup of black beans, drained
- 3 cups of kale
- 1 ½ cups of shredded cheddar cheese
- salt & pepper to taste

**Directions:**

1. Place a large skillet over medium-high heat and drizzle a little oil to lightly coat the surface of the pan.

2. Add the onions, mixed herb spice and pepper into the skillet and fry for 2 minutes until the onions have softened.

3. Add the ground beef, garlic paste, and a pinch of salt and pepper into the skillet. Mix the contents up, crumbling the beef while you stir. Continue stirring the mix until the beef has browned and the juices have evaporated (for about 8 minutes).

4. Lower the heat and add the canned tomatoes and black beans into the skillet. Mix once more, then add the kale into the mix. Let the mixture simmer for another 5 minutes.

5. Sprinkle the shredded cheese over the top of the dish and allow it to melt (about 2-3 more minutes).

6. Serve the dish with some lettuce & sliced avocado.

**Nutrition** 341 Calories 20g Fat 30g Protein

# Cheese Taco Shells

Preparation Time: 10 minutes

Cooking Time: 10 minutes

Servings: 4

**Ingredients:**

- ¼ cup of ground beef
- 2 tbsps. of oil
- ½ tsp of garlic paste
- 6 slices of preferred cheese
- 2 tomatoes, diced
- 3 tbsps. of diced red onion
- ½ jalapeno, diced
- 1 lime's worth of juice
- 2 tbsps. of cilantro
- 1 tsp of mixed herb spice
- salt & pepper to taste
- sour cream for topping

**Directions:**

1. Preheat the oven to 375°F and place a skillet on medium-high heat.

2. Drizzle the oil into the skillet and add the onion, ground beef, mixed herb spice, tomatoes, garlic paste, salt, and pepper into the skillet. Fry for 5 minutes, while stirring regularly. Once the beef has crumbled and is browned, remove the pan from the heat.

3. Place each slice of cheese into a cup of a muffin tray and place it in the oven for 5 minutes. Remove the tray from

---

the oven and leave the cheese in the muffin cups to cool down and harden.

4. Carefully remove the cheese cups from the muffin cup holders.
5. Add the jalapeno, cilantro and lime juice into the beef mixture once it has cooled down, and mix the ingredients together.
6. Spoon the mixture evenly into the cheese cups and add a dollop of cream cheese to the top of each cup.

**Nutrition** 264 Calories 22g Fat 13g Protein

# Pork Rind Tortillas

Preparation Time: 10 minutes

Cooking Time: 20 minutes

Servings: 12

**Ingredients:**

- 4 oz of cooked pork rinds
- 8 oz of softened cream cheese
- 8 eggs
- 1 tbsps. of garlic powder
- 1 tbsp of cumin powder
- salt & pepper to taste
- ½ red bell pepper, sliced thinly
- 1 scallion, chopped thinly
- 1/3 cup of shredded mozzarella
- 1 lime's worth of juice

**Directions:**

1. Add the pork rinds into a food processor and a pinch of pepper. Pulse the ingredients for about 10-15 seconds until the mixture is fine. Remove the contents from the processor and set it aside.

2. Add the cream cheese, eggs, garlic powder and cumin into the food processor, along with a pinch of salt. Pulse the contents for 40 seconds until it forms a smooth texture.

3. Place a saucepan/skillet on the stove and bring the heat to a medium-high. Coat the surface with some cooking spray or coconut oil.

4. Dollop the egg batter onto the pan and spread the dollops out as thin as possible. Fry both sides of the tortilla for 1 minute, until the sides are both a golden brown.

5. Fill the tortillas with a spoonful of the pork rind, then add in a few bell peppers slices, a few scallion slices and a sprinkle of mozzarella. Drizzle lime juice over the top and a dash of hot sauce if preferred.

**Nutrition** 170 Calories 13g Fat 12g Protein

# Mushroom Masala

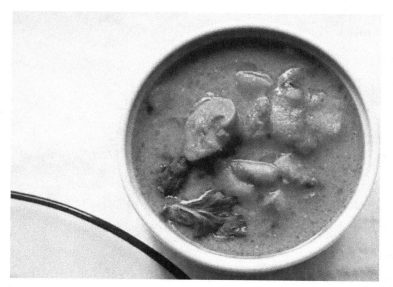

Preparation Time: 15 minutes

Cooking Time: 15 minutes

Servings: 4

**Ingredients:**

- 10 cashew nuts
- 2 cups of mushrooms, sliced
- ½ cup of peas
- 1 tbsp of ginger and garlic paste
- 1 chili
- 1 ½ cups of diced tomato
- ½ tsp of garam masala
- ¼ tsp of turmeric
- 1 tsp of coriander powder
- 1 tsp of cumin

- 1 ½ tsps. of fenugreek
- 2 tbsps. of chopped cilantro
- ½ lemon's worth of juice
- cauliflower rice for serving (optional)

**Directions:**

1. Add the cashew nuts into a small bowl filled with water, and soak the cashews for 15 minutes. Once soaked, drain the nuts and add it into a food processor with ¼ cup of water. Blend the mixture into a smooth puree.
2. Set the nut puree aside, then add the onions, tomatoes, ginger and garlic paste and the chili into a blender. Blend this mixture into a smooth puree and set it aside.
3. Prepare the instant pot and add in the oil, cumin, coriander, turmeric and garam masala into the pot. Sauté the spices for a few seconds, then add the tomato puree into the pot.
4. Cook the mixture for 4 minutes, stirring slowly.
5. Add the mushrooms, peas and ½ a cup of water into the pot and stir once more. Close the lid of the pot and pressure cook on high pressure for 3 minutes.
6. Release the pressure naturally for about 5 minutes, then quick release.
7. Pour the cashew nut mixture into the pot, along with the fenugreek and lemon juice. Mix the contents well for about 3 minutes, until the curry starts to thicken.
8. Serve with cauliflower rice, or enjoy it on its own!

**Nutrition** 180 Calories 9g Fat 6g Protein

# Beef and Eggplant Kebab

Preparation Time: 20 minutes

Cooking Time: 15 minutes

Serving: 4

## Ingredients:

- 3 tbsp oil
- 1/2 tsp dried thyme
- 1/2 tsp oregano
- 2 eggs (beaten)
- 1/2 eggplant
- 1/2 tsp chili pepper (ground)
- 1/4 cup olive oil
- 4 garlic cloves (crushed)
- 1 cup parsley leaves (chopped)
- 1 lb. beef (minced)
- 1 tsp salt
- 1/2 tsp black pepper

## Directions:

1. Cut the eggplant into thin slices of about half inch. Season with salt and set aside. Put minced meat in a large bowl, add thyme, eggs, chili pepper, onions, parsley, olive oil, garlic, salt, oregano, and black pepper. Combine the mixture. Shape equal-sized patties with wet hands. Preheat a skillet over medium-high heat and grease with oil. Rinse the eggplant slices sprinkled with salt and pat dry with hand or paper towel. Thread eggplant slices and

patties alternately onto skewers and place on the preheated skillet. Flip the sides occasionally and cook for 15 minutes. Remove from the heat and garnish with parsley. Serve warm with low-carb pita bread.

**Nutrition** 371 Calories 24g Fat 34g Protein

# Six-Ingredient Pizza

Preparation Time: 10 minutes

Cooking Time: 10 minutes

Servings: 1

## Ingredients:

- 1 ½ cups of shredded mozzarella cheese
- 2 tbsps. of cream cheese, cubed
- 2 eggs
- 1/3 cup of coconut/almond flour
- ¼ cup of pepperoni slices
- ½ tsp of mixed herbs
- a handful of rockets

## Directions:

1. Preheat the 425°F and line a baking tray with parchment paper.
2. In a large bowl, add the mozzarella and cream cheese into the bowl and place it in the microwave for about 40 seconds, then stir the mixture with a fork and place it back in the microwave for another 40 seconds.
3. In a separate bowl, crack the eggs and beat them into a light, fluffy mixture. Pour the beaten eggs and flour into the bowl with the cheese and mix it together, using your hands to knead the dough.
4. Roll the dough ball out onto the baking tray and use a rolling pin to roll the dough to 1/3" in thickness.

5. Poke a few holes in the dough using a toothpick/fork, so that the dough doesn't bubble while baking.
6. Place the pizza in the oven for 6 minutes, then remove.
7. If there are any bubbles that are forming, poke holes in the bubbles to deflate them.
8. Layer on a few slices of pepperoni onto the pizza and sprinkle on the mixed herb spice. Place the tray back in the oven for 5 more minutes.
9. Lay a few rocket leaves on top of the pizza and serve warm.

**Nutrition** 483 Calories 27g Fat 30g Protein 13g

# APPETIZER RECIPES

## Panda Express® Chicken Pot Stickers

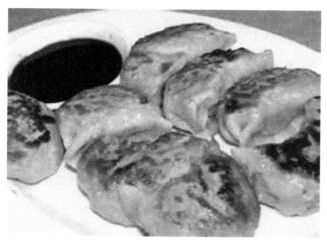

Preparation Time: 40 minutes

Cooking Time: 30 minutes

Servings: 50

**Ingredients:**

- 1/2 cup + 2 tablespoons soy sauce, divided
- 1 tablespoon rice vinegar
- 3 tablespoons chives, divided
- 1 tablespoon sesame seeds
- 1 teaspoon sriracha hot sauce
- 1-pound ground pork
- 3 cloves garlic, minced
- 1 egg, beaten

- 1 1/2 tablespoons sesame oil
- 1 tablespoon fresh ginger, minced
- 50 dumpling wrappers
- 1 cup vegetable oil, for frying
- 1-quart water

**Directions:**

1. In a mixing bowl, whisk together the 1/2 cup of soy sauce, vinegar, and 1 tablespoon of the chives, sesame seeds and sriracha to make the dipping sauce. In a separate bowl, mix together the pork, garlic, egg, the rest of the chives, the 2 tablespoons of soy sauce, sesame oil and the ginger. Add 1 tablespoon of filling to each dumpling wrapper. Pinch the sides of the wrappers together to seal. You may need to wet the edges a bit, so they'll stick.

2. Heat the cup of oil in a large skillet. When hot, working in batches, add the dumplings and cook until golden brown on all sides. Take care of not overloading your pan. Add the water and cook until tender, then serve with the dipping sauce.

**Nutrition:** Calories 260; Fat 6g; Carbs 39g; Protein 13g

# Panda Express® Cream Cheese Rangoon

Preparation Time: 5 minutes
Cooking Time: 5 minutes

Servings: 24 minutes

**Ingredients:**

- 24 wonton wrappers
- 1/2-pound cream cheese, softened
- 1/4 cup green onions, chopped
- 1/2 teaspoon salt
- 1/2 teaspoon garlic powder
- Oil for frying

**Directions:**

1. Add the cream cheese, green onions, garlic powder and salt to a medium sized bowl and then mix it well. Lay wonton wrappers out and then moisten the edges of the first one. Add about 1/2 tablespoon of filling to the center of the wrapper and seal it by pinching the edges together, starting with the corners and working your way inward. Make sure to seal tightly. Repeat this with the remaining wrappers. Next, add about 3 inches of oil to a pot. Heat it for about 350°F, then add the wontons a few at a time and cook until brown. Remove from oil and place on a paper-towel-lined plate to drain.

**Nutrition:** Calories 193; Fat 8g; Carbs 24g; Protein 5g

# Panda Express® Chicken Egg Roll

Preparation Time: 10 minutes
Cooking Time: 5 minutes
Servings: 6-8

## Ingredients:

- 2 tablespoons soy sauce, divided
- 2 cloves garlic, minced, divided
- 2 green onions, chopped, divided
- 3 tablespoons vegetable oil, divided
- 1/2-pound boneless skinless chicken breasts, cooked whole & cut in pieces
- 1/2 head green cabbage, thinly shredded
- 1 large carrot, peeled and shredded1 cup bean sprouts
- 12-16 egg roll wrappers
- 1 tablespoon cornstarch mixed with 3 tablespoons water
- Peanut Oil for frying

## Directions:

1. In a resalable plastic bag, combine 1 tablespoon of the soy sauce with 1 clove of minced garlic, 1 green onion, and 1 tablespoon of the oil. Mix well. Add the cut-up chicken pieces, seal the bag, and squish it around to make sure the chicken is covered. Refrigerate for at least 30 minutes.

2. After the chicken has marinated, pour 1 tablespoon of the oil into a large skillet and heat over medium-high heat. When the oil is hot, add the chicken and cook, stirring occasionally, until the chicken is cooked through. Remove the chicken from the skillet and set aside. Pour the remaining tablespoon of oil into the skillet and add the cabbage, carrots and remaining soy sauce. Cook and stir until the carrots and cabbage start to soften, then add

the bean sprouts and the remaining garlic and green onions. Cook another minute or so.

3. Drain the chicken and vegetables thoroughly using either cheesecloth or a mesh strainer. Getting all the excess liquid out will keep the egg rolls from getting soggy. In a Dutch oven or large sauce pan heat 3 inches of oil to 375°F. Place about 2 tablespoons of the chicken and vegetables into the center of each egg roll wrapper. Fold the ends up and roll up to cover the filling. Seal by dipping your finger in the water and cornstarch mixture and covering the edges.

4. Cook the egg rolls in batches, a few at a time, for about five minutes or until golden brown and crispy. Remove from oil to a paper-towel-lined plate to drain.

**Nutrition:** Calories 349; Fat 4g; Carbs 176g; Protein 13 g

# Panda Express® Veggie Spring Roll

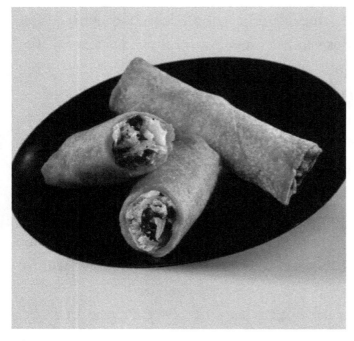

Preparation Time: 15 minutes

Cooking Time: 5 minutes

Servings: 6-8

## Ingredients:

- 4 teaspoons vegetable oil, divided
- 3 eggs, beaten
- 1 medium head cabbage, finely shredded
- 1/2 carrots, julienned
- 1 (8-ounce) can shredded bamboo shoots
- 1 cup dried, shredded wood ear mushroom, rehydrated

- 1-pound Chinese barbecue or roasted pork, cut into matchsticks
- 1/2 cup chopped Chinese yellow chives
- 1 green onion, thinly sliced
- 2 1/2 teaspoons soy sauce
- 1 teaspoon salt
- 1 teaspoon sugar
- 1 (14-ounce) package egg roll wrappers
- 1 egg white, beaten
- 1-quart oil for frying, or as needed

**Directions:**

1. Heat 1 tablespoon of oil over medium-high heat in a large skillet.

2. When the skillet is hot, add the beaten eggs and cook until firm, then flip and cook a bit longer like an omelet. When set, remove from the pan. Cut into strips and set aside.

3. Add the remaining oil to the skillet and heat. When hot, add the cabbage and carrot and cook for a couple of minutes until they start to soften. Then add the bamboo shoots, mushrooms, pork, green onions, chives, soy sauce, salt and sugar. Cook until the veggies are soft, then stir in the egg. Transfer the mixture to a bowl and refrigerate for about 1 hour.

4. When cooled, add about 2-3 tablespoons of filling to each egg roll wrapper. Brush some of the beaten egg around the edges of the wrapper and roll up, tucking in the ends first.

5. When all of the wrappers are filled, heat about 6 inches of oil to 350°F in a deep saucepan, Dutch oven or fryer.

6. Add egg rolls to the hot oil a couple at a time, remove from oil to a paper-towel-lined plate to drain when golden brown and crispy.

7. Serve with chili sauce or sweet and sour sauce.

**Nutrition:** Calories 132; Fat 3.3g; Carbs 5.5g; Protein 32g

# PF Chang® Hot and Sour Soup

Preparation Time: 10 minutes

Cooking Time: 10 minutes

Servings: 4-6

**Ingredients:**

- 1-quart chicken stock
- 6 ounces of chicken breasts cut into thin strips
- 1/2 cup cornstarch
- 1 cup soy sauce
- 1 teaspoon white pepper
- 6 ounces wood ear mushrooms cut into strips or canned straw mushrooms, if wood ear can't be found
- 1/2 cup water
- 2 eggs, beaten
- 1/2 cup white vinegar
- 1 (6 ounce) can bamboo shoots, cut into strips
- 6 ounces silken tofu, cut into strips
- Sliced green onions for garnish

**Directions:**

1. Cook the chicken strips in a hot skillet until cooked through. Set aside.
2. Add the chicken stock, soy sauce, pepper and bamboo shoots to a stockpot and bring to a boil. Stir in the chicken and let cook for about 3-4 minutes.
3. In a small dish, make slurry with the cornstarch and water. Add a bit at a time to the stockpot until the broth thickens to your desired consistency.

4. Stir in the beaten eggs and cook for about 45 seconds or until the eggs are done.
5. Remove from the heat and add the vinegar and tofu. Garnish with sliced green onions.

**Nutrition:** Calories 345; Fat 1.2g; Carbs 2.2g; Protein 23.3g

# PF Chang® Lettuce Wraps

Preparation Time: 10 minutes

Cooking Time: 10 minutes

Servings: 4

**Ingredients:**

- 1 tablespoon olive oil
- 1-pound ground chicken
- 2 cloves garlic, minced
- 1 onion, diced
- 1/4 cup hoisin sauce
- 2 tablespoons soy sauce
- 1 (8-ounce) can of whole water chestnuts, drained and diced
- 1 tablespoon rice wine vinegar
- 2 green onions, thinly sliced
- 1 tablespoon Sriracha (optional)
- 1 tablespoon ginger, freshly grated
- 1 head iceberg lettuce
- Kosher salt and freshly ground black pepper to taste

**Directions:**

1. Add the oil to a deep skillet or saucepan and heat over medium-high heat. Add the chicken when hot and cook until it is completely cooked through. Stir while cooking to make sure it is properly crumbled.

2. Drain any excess fat from the skillet, and then add the garlic, onion, hoisin sauce, soy sauce, ginger, sriracha and vinegar.
3. Cook it until the onions have softened, then stir in the water chestnuts and green onion and cook for another minute or so.
4. Add salt and pepper to taste. Serve with lettuce leaves and eat by wrapping them up like a taco.

**Nutrition:** Calories 560; Fat 29g; Carbs 51g; Protein 23g

# PF Chang® Shrimp Dumplings

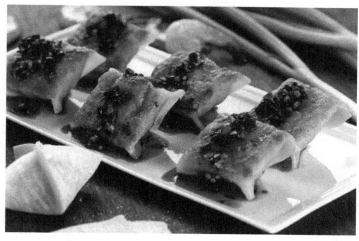

Preparation Time: 20 minutes

Cooking Time: 10 minutes

Servings: 4-6

## Ingredients:

- 1-pound medium shrimp, peeled, deveined, washed and dried, divided
- 2 tablespoons carrot, finely minced
- 2 tablespoons green onion, finely minced
- 1 teaspoon ginger, freshly minced
- 2 tablespoons oyster sauce
- 1/4 teaspoon sesame oil
- 1 package wonton wrappers

Sauce

- 1 cup soy sauce
- 2 tablespoons white vinegar

- 1/2 teaspoon chili paste
- 2 tablespoons granulated sugar
- 1/2 teaspoon ginger, freshly minced
- Sesame oil to taste
- 1 cup water
- 1 tablespoon cilantro leaves

**Directions:**
1. Finely mince 1/2 pound of the shrimp in a food processor or blender. Dice the other 1/2 pound of shrimp. In a mixing bowl, combine both the minced and diced shrimp with the remaining ingredients. Spoon about 1 teaspoon of the mixture into each wonton wrapper. Wet the edges of the wrapper with your finger, then fold up and seal tightly.
2. Cover and then refrigerate it for at least an hour. In a medium bowl, combine all of the ingredients for the sauce and stir until well combined. When ready to serve, boil water in a saucepan and cover with a steamer. You may want to lightly oil the steamer to keep the dumplings from sticking. Steam the dumplings for 7-10 minutes. Serve with sauce.

**Nutrition:** Calories 244; Fat 20g; Carbs 57g; Protein 63g

# DESSERT RECIPES

## Maple Butter Blondie

Preparation Time: 15 minutes
Cooking Time: 35 minutes
Servings: 9

**Ingredients**

- 1/3 cup butter, melted
- 1 cup brown sugar, packed
- 1 large egg, beaten
- 1 tablespoon vanilla extract
- ½ teaspoon baking powder
- 1/8 teaspoon baking soda
- 1/8 teaspoon salt
- 1 cup flour
- 2/3 cup white chocolate chips
- 1/3 cup pecans, chopped (or walnuts)

Maple butter sauce

- ¾ cup maple syrup
- 8 oz. cream cheese room temp
- ½ cup butter
- ¾ cup brown sugar
- ¼ cup pecans, chopped
- Vanilla ice cream, for serving

**Direction:**

1. Prep the oven to 350°F and brush a 9x9 baking pan with cooking spray.

2. In a mixing bowl, combine the butter, brown sugar, egg, and vanilla, and beat until smooth. Incorporate the baking powder, baking soda, salt, and flour, and stir until it is well incorporated. Fold in the white chocolate chips.

3. Bake for 20–25 minutes. Prep maple butter sauce by combining the maple syrup and butter in a medium saucepan.

4. Cook at low heat until the butter melts. Add the brown sugar and cream cheese. Stir constantly until the cream cheese has completely melted, then remove the pot from the heat. Pull out the blondies from the oven and cut them into squares.

5. Top with vanilla ice cream, maple butter sauce, and chopped nuts.

**Nutrition:** 40g Carbohydrates 14g fats 3g protein

# Apple Chimi Cheesecake

Preparation Time: 10 minutes

Cooking Time: 10 minutes

Servings: 2

**Ingredients**

- 2 (9 inch) flour tortillas
- ¼ cup granulated sugar
- ½ teaspoon cinnamon
- 3 ounces cream cheese, softened
- ½ teaspoon vanilla extract
- 1/3 cup apple
- Oil for frying
- Vanilla ice cream (optional)
- Caramel topping (optional)

**Directions**

1. Make sure your tortillas and cream cheese are at room temperature; this will make them both easier to work with. Mix sugar and cinnamon.
2. Scourge cream cheese and vanilla until smooth. Fold in the apple. Divide the apple and cheese mixture in two and place half in the center of each tortilla. Set aside least an inch margin around the outside.
3. Fold the tortilla top to the middle, then the bottom to the middle, and then roll it up from the sides. Cook about half an inch of oil in a skillet over medium heat.
4. Place the filled tortillas into the skillet and fry on each side until they are golden brown. Situate them to a paper

towel lined plate to drain any excess oil, then immediately coat them with the cinnamon and sugar. Serve with a scoop of ice cream.

**Nutrition:** 43g Carbohydrates 12g fats 5g protein

# Triple Chocolate Meltdown

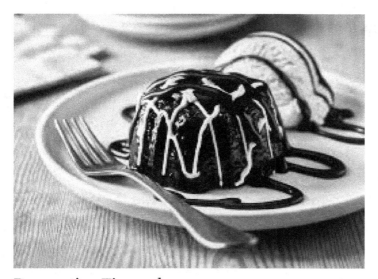

Preparation Time: 1 hour

Cooking Time: 30 minutes

Servings: 8

## Ingredients

- 2 cups heavy cream, divided
- 1 cup white chocolate chips
- 1 cup semi-sweet chocolate chips
- 1-pound bittersweet chocolate, chopped
- ½ cup butter, softened
- 6 eggs
- 1 ½ cups of sugar
- 1 ½ cups all-purpose flour
- Ice cream, for serving

## Directions

1. Preheat the oven to 400°F.

2. Prepare 8 ramekins by first coating the inside with butter then sprinkling them with flour so the bottom and sides are covered. Place them on a baking tray.

3. In a saucepan, bring 1 cup of heavy cream to a simmer. Remove it from the heat and add the white chocolate chips, stirring until the chocolate is melted and the mixture is smooth. Allow it to cool for about a half an hour, stirring occasionally.

4. Repeat with the other cup of cream and the semi-sweet chocolate chips. In a double boiler, combine the bittersweet chocolate with the softened butter and stir until the chocolate is melted and the mixture is smooth. Remove the bowl from the heat and allow it to cool for about 10 minutes

5. In a mixing bowl, beat the eggs and the sugar together for about 2 minutes, or until the mixture is foamy. Use a rubber spatula to fold in the bittersweet chocolate mixture. Turn the mixer to low and beat in the flour half a cup at a time, being careful not to overmix the batter.

6. Pour the batter evenly into the prepared ramekins and place the baking tray in oven. Bake for about 18 minutes. When done, the cakes should have a slight crust but still be soft in the middle. Remove them from oven when they have reached this look. If you cook them too long you won't get the lava cake effect.

7. Let the ramekins sit on the tray for 2–3 minutes and then invert them onto serving plates. Drizzle some of both the

semi-sweet and white chocolate sauces over the top and
serve with a scoop of ice cream.

**Nutrition:** 39g carbohydrates 15g fats 6g protein

# Chocolate Mousse Dessert Shooter

Preparation Time: 30 minutes

Cooking Time: 0 minute

Serving: 4

## Ingredients

- 2 tablespoons butter
- 6 ounces semi-sweet chocolate chips (1 cup), divided
- 1 teaspoon vanilla
- 2 eggs, separated, at room temperature
- 2 tablespoons sugar
- ½ cup heavy cream
- 8 Oreo® cookies
- ½ cup prepared fudge sauce
- Canned whipped cream

## Directions

1. Melt the butter and all but 1 tablespoon of the chocolate chips in a double boiler. When they are melted, stir in the vanilla and remove from the heat. Whisk in the egg yolks.

2. Beat the egg whites until they form soft peaks, and then fold them into the chocolate mixture. Beat the sugar and heavy cream in a separate bowl until it forms stiff peaks or is the consistency that you desire. Fold this into the chocolate mixture.

3. Crush the remaining chocolate chips into small pieces and stir them into the chocolate. Crush the Oreos. (You

can either scrape out the cream from the cookies or just crush the entire cookie.)

4. Spoon the cookie crumbs into the bottom of your cup and pat them down. Layer the chocolate mixture on top. Finish with whipped cream and either more chocolate chips or Oreo mixture. Store in the refrigerator until ready to serve.

**Nutrition:** 45g carbohydrates 12g fats 5g protein

# Deadly Chocolate Sin

Preparation Time: 12 minutes

Cooking Time: 10 minutes

Servings: 12

**Ingredients**

- 1-2 tablespoons butter for greasing or cooking spray
- 6 ounces semisweet chocolate
- 1 cup unsalted butter
- 1 teaspoon vanilla extract
- 4 eggs, at room temperature
- 4 egg yolks, at room temperature
- ½ cup brown sugar, firmly packed
- 6 tablespoons cornstarch
- 1 (10 ounce) package frozen raspberries in heavy syrup, thawed
- 1-pint fresh raspberries
- 2 ounces bitter chocolate
- 12 triangular cookies or chocolate pieces
- 12 sprigs fresh mint

**Directions**

1. Preheat the oven to 375°F. Prepare 12 (4 ounce) ramekins by buttering or spraying them with non-stick cooking spray. Combine the chocolate, unsalted butter, and vanilla in a double boiler and melt the chocolate, stirring to combine. In a large mixing bowl, beat together the eggs, egg yolks, and brown sugar. Mix this

on high for 5–7 minutes, or until the volume almost doubles.

2. Set the mixer to low and add the cornstarch one tablespoon at a time, beating after each addition. Turn the mixer back to high and beat another 5 minutes or until soft peaks form.

3. Now, fold the chocolate into the egg mixture, making sure to scrape the bottom and sides of the bowl.

4. Pour the batter into the prepared ramekins and bake for 10 minutes. After 10 minutes, remove the ramekins from the oven and allow them to cool. Store in the refrigerator, covered with plastic wrap, until ready to serve.

5. When ready to serve, run a knife around the edges to loosen the cake, then invert the cake on serving plates.

6. Purée the thawed raspberries in a blender, then ladle them over the top of each cake. Top with fresh raspberries, chocolate pieces, and mint. Serve

**Nutrition:** 40g carbohydrates 10g fats 6g protein

# Orange Creamsicle Cake

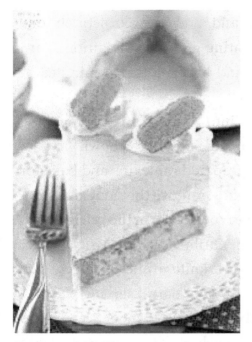

Preparation Time: 30 minutes

Cooking Time: 35–45 minutes

Serving: 8 - 10

**Ingredients**

- 1 (18.25 ounce) box orange cake mix
- 1 (3 ounce) package orange-flavored gelatin
- 1 cup boiling water
- 1 (3.4 ounce) package instant vanilla pudding mix
- 1 cup milk
- 1 teaspoon vanilla extract
- 1 teaspoon orange extract
- 1 (8 ounce) tub Cool Whip®, thawed

- White chocolate shavings, to garnish

**Directions**

1. Preheat the oven to 350°F and prepare two 9-inch round cake pans by greasing and dusting them with flour. In a large bowl, prepare the packaged cake mix according to the package directions. Divide the batter evenly between the prepared cake pans.

2. Bake for 35–45 minutes, or until a toothpick inserted in the center comes out clean. Remove the cakes from the oven. While they are still hot, use the handle end of a wooden spoon to poke holes throughout.

3. Prepare the gelatin with one cup of hot water, and when it is dissolved completely, pour it over the hot cake, making sure the gelatin goes into all the holes.

4. Let the cake sit and cool completely. (You can put it in the refrigerator to speed up the process if you like.) Prepare the vanilla pudding using only one cup of milk. Fold in the Cool Whip, making sure it is well incorporated.

5. Put a layer of the pudding mixture between the cake layers and use the remaining to completely frost the cake. Garnish with chocolate shavings and grated orange peel if desired. Refrigerate until ready to serve.

**Nutrition:** 41g carbohydrates 12g fats 3g protein

# Cinnamon Apple Turnover

Preparation Time: 10 minutes

Cooking Time: 25 minutes

Servings: 4 - 6

**Ingredients**

- 1 large Granny Smith apple, peeled, cored, and diced
- ½ teaspoon cornstarch
- ¼ teaspoon cinnamon
- Dash ground nutmeg
- ¼ cup brown sugar
- ¼ cup applesauce
- ¼ teaspoon vanilla extract
- 1 tablespoon butter, melted
- 1 sheet of puff pastry, thawed
- Whipped cream or vanilla ice cream, to serve

**Directions**

1. Preheat the oven to 400°F. Prepare a baking sheet by spraying it with non-stick cooking spray or using a bit of oil on a paper towel.

2. In a mixing bowl, mix together the apples, cornstarch, cinnamon, nutmeg, and brown sugar. Stir to make sure the apples are well covered with the spices. Then stir in the applesauce and the vanilla.

3. Lay out your puff pastry and cut it into squares. You should be able to make 4 or 6 depending on how big you want your turnovers to be and how big your pastry is.

4. Place some of the apple mixture in the center of each square and fold the corners of the pastry up to make a pocket. Pinch the edges together to seal. Then brush a bit of the melted butter over the top to give the turnovers that nice brown color.

5. Place the filled pastry onto the prepared baking pan and transfer to the preheated oven. Bake 20–25 minutes, or until they become a golden brown in color. Serve with whipped cream or vanilla ice cream.

**Nutrition:** 43g carbohydrates 13g fats 4g protein

# Burger King's Hershey's Sundae Pie

Preparation Time: 20 minutes

Cooking Time: 10 minutes

Servings: 8

**Ingredients**

Crust

- 1½ cups crushed chocolate wafers
- 2 tablespoons sugar
- ½ cup melted butter
- Cream cheese layer
- 8 ounces cream cheese
- ¾ cup powdered sugar
- 8 ounces Cool Whip or cream, plus more for topping
- 1 teaspoon vanilla extract

Chocolate layer

- 1 (3½-ounce) box chocolate pudding
- 1½ cups milk
- Chocolate syrup, for drizzling
- Chocolate chips, for topping

**Directions:**

1. Preheat oven to 350°F. Meanwhile, prepare the crust. Place ingredients in food processor or blender and pulse until well-blended. Spread and press into a 9-inch pie pan. Bake until fragrant and set (about 10 minutes). Place on wire rack to cool.

2. Prepare the cream cheese layer. Beat the cream cheese until softened. Beat in sugar, Cool Whip and vanilla until well-blended. Spread evenly over cooled crust.

3. Use 1½ cups milk to prepare pudding (follow packaging instructions) and spread over cream filling.

4. Top with dollops of Cool Whip, drizzle with chocolate syrup and sprinkle with chocolate chips.

5. Let chill to set.

**Nutrition:** 420 Calories 27.8g Total Fat 5.2g Protein

# MEXICAN RECIPES

## Fajita Burgers

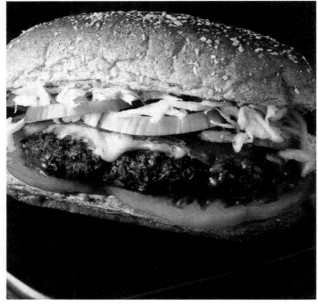

Preparation Time: 15 mins

Cooking Time: 25 mins

Servings: 4

**Ingredients:**

- 1/4 C. tomatillo salsa
- 2 tsp fajita seasoning mix, divided
- 2 tbsp. avocados, chopped
- 1/4 tsp salt, divided
- 1 tbsp. fresh cilantro, chopped

- 1 tbsp. tomato paste
- 2 slices white bread
- 1 lb. ground turkey
- 1/2 C. onion, finely chopped
- 1 egg white
- 1/2 C. red bell pepper, finely chopped
- 4 whole wheat hamburger buns, toasted
- 1/2 C. green bell pepper, finely chopped

**Directions:**

1. In a small bowl, mix together the tomatillo salsa, avocado and cilantro and keep aside.
2. In a food processor, place the bread slices and pulse till a coarse crumb forms measure 1 C
3. Grease a large nonstick skillet with the nonstick spray and heat on medium-high heat.
4. Add the onion and bell peppers and sauté for about 5 minutes.
5. Stir in 1/2 tsp of the fajita seasoning and 1/8 tsp of the salt.
6. Remove from the heat and keep aside to cool.
7. In a large bowl, add 1 C. of the breadcrumbs, onion mixture, remaining 1 1/2 tsp of the fajita seasoning, remaining 1/8 tsp of the salt, tomato paste, turkey and egg white and mix till well combined.
8. With damp hands, divide the turkey mixture into 4 (3/4-inch thick) patties.
9. Grease the same skillet with the nonstick spray and heat on medium heat.

10. Add patties and cook for about 4 minutes per side.
11. 1Place 1 patty on bottom half of each bun and top with 1 1/2 tbsp. of the salsa mixture.
12. 1Cover with the remaining half of the bun.

**Nutrition:** Calories 351.0Fat 12.8gCholesterol 78.3mgSodium 520.1mg

Carbohydrates 30.8gProtein 29.1g

# Spicy Mexican Quinoa

Preparation Time: 20 mins

Cooking Time: 40 mins

Servings: 4

**Ingredients:**

- 1 tbsp. olive oil
- 1 C. quinoa, rinsed
- chili peppers
- 1 small onion, chopped
- 1 envelope taco seasoning mix
- 2 cloves garlic, minced
- 2 C. low-sodium chicken broth
- 1 jalapeno pepper, seeded and chopped
- 1/4 C. chopped fresh cilantro
- 1 (10 oz.) can diced tomatoes with green

**Directions:**

1. In a large skillet, heat the oil on medium heat and stir fry the quinoa and onion for about 5 minutes.
2. Add the garlic and jalapeño pepper and cook for about 1-2 minutes.
3. Stir in the undrained can have diced tomatoes with green chilis, taco seasoning mix and chicken broth and bring to a boil.
4. Reduce the heat to medium-low and simmer for about 15-20 minutes.
5. Stir in cilantro and serve.

**Nutrition:** Calories 244 kcal Fat 6.1 g Carbohydrates 38.1g Protein 8.1 g Cholesterol 2 mg Sodium 986 mg

# South of the Border Pesto

Preparation Time: 10 mins

Cooking Time: 10 mins

Servings: 6

**Ingredients:**

- 1/4 C. hulled pumpkin seeds (pepitas)
- 1 serrano chili pepper, seeded
- 1 bunch cilantro
- 1/2 tsp salt
- 1/4 C. grated cotija cheese
- 6 tbsp. olive oil
- 4 cloves garlic

**Directions:**

1. In a food processor, add the pumpkin seeds and pulse till chopped roughly.
2. Add the remaining ingredients and pulse till smooth.

**Nutrition:** Calories 176 kcal Fat 17.8 g Cholesterol 2.4g Sodium 2.9 g Carbohydrates 6 mg Protein 262 mg

# El Pollo Soup

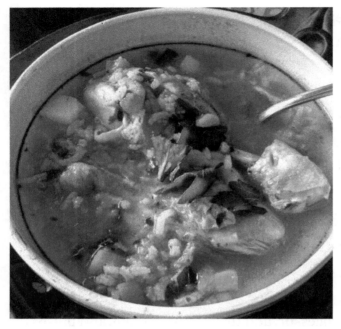

Preparation Time: 20 mins

Cooking Time: 1 h 5 mins

Servings: 4

**Ingredients:**

- 3 cooked, boneless chicken breast halves,
- shredded
- 1/2 green bell pepper, chopped
- 1 (15 oz.) can kidney beans
- 1/2 red bell pepper, chopped
- 1 C. whole kernel corn
- 1 (4 oz.) can chopped green chili peppers
- 1 (14.5 oz.) can stewed tomatoes
- 2 (14.5 oz.) cans chicken broth

- 1/2 C. chopped onion
- 1 tbsp. ground cumin

**Directions:**

1. In a large pan mix together all the ingredients on medium heat.
2. Simmer for about 45 minutes.

**Nutrition:** Calories 335 kcal Fat 7.7 g Carbohydrates 37.7g Protein 31.5 g Cholesterol 62 mg Sodium 841 mg

# Restaurant-Style Latin Rice

Preparation Time: 20 mins

Cooking Time: 55 mins

Servings: 6

**Ingredients:**

- 1 lb. lean ground beef
- 1/2 tsp chili powder
- 1 onion, diced
- 1/2 tsp paprika
- 1 green bell pepper, diced
- 1/2 tsp garlic powder
- 1 (14 oz.) can beef broth
- 1/2 tsp salt
- 2 C. fresh corn kernels
- 1/2 tsp ground black pepper
- 1 (10 oz.) can diced tomatoes with green
- 1 tsp minced cilantro
- chili peppers
- 1 1/2 C. uncooked white rice
- 1 (15 oz.) can tomato sauce
- 1 C. shredded Cheddar cheese
- 1/2 C. salsa

**Directions:**

1. Heat a medium pan on medium heat and cook the beef till browned completely.
2. Drain off the grease from the pan.

3. Add the onion and green pepper and cook till the onion becomes tender.
4. Stir in the beef broth, corn, tomatoes with green chili peppers and tomato sauce, salsa, chili powder, paprika, garlic powder, salt, pepper and cilantro and bring to a boil.
5. Stir in the rice and cook, covered for about 25 minutes.
6. Top with the Cheddar cheese and cook for about 10 minutes.

**Nutrition**: Calories 510 kcal Fat 18.3 g Carbohydrates 59.1g Protein 28.3 g Cholesterol 74 mg Sodium 1294 mg

# Canela Brownies

Preparation Time: 20 mins
Cooking Time: 1 h 10 mins
Servings: per Recipe: 30

## Ingredients:
- 1 1/2 C. unsalted butter
- 3 C. white sugar
- 1 3/4 tsp ground Mexican cinnamon (canela)
- 6 eggs
- 1/2 tsp ground pequin chili pepper
- 1 tbsp. vanilla extract
- 3/4 tsp kosher salt
- 1 1/4 C. unsweetened cocoa powder
- 3/4 tsp baking powder
- 1 1/2 C. all-purpose flour

## Directions:
1. Set your oven to 350 degrees F before doing anything else and line a 15x12-inch baking dish with the parchment paper, leaving about 3 inches of paper overhanging 2 sides to use as handles.
2. In a microwave-safe bowl, add the butter and microwave on Medium for about 1 minute.
3. Add the sugar and mix till well combined.
4. Add the eggs, one at a time, and mix till well combined.
5. Stir in the vanilla extract.

6. In a bowl, sift together the flour, cocoa, cinnamon, pequin pepper, salt and baking powder.
7. Add the flour mixture into the butter mixture and mix till well combined.
8. Transfer the mixture into the prepared baking dish evenly.
9. Cook in the oven for about 20-25 minutes or till a toothpick inserted into the center comes out clean.
10. Remove from the oven and keep aside to cool in the pan.
11. Remove the parchment paper handles to remove the brownies for slicing.

**Nutrition:** Calories 206 kcal Fat 10.8 g Carbohydrates 27g Protein 2.7 g Cholesterol 62 mg Sodium 76 mg

# CONCLUSION

Copycat recipes are the best thing to happen to cooking since the invention of the pressure cooker. I love copycat recipes because they allow me to make something delicious, but in a fraction of the time it takes me to make it from scratch. Copycat recipes are a great way to save money and time. You don't have to rely on specialty ingredients that you may not have access to, or ingredients that you don't know how to use.

Copycat recipes are a great way to make money. It's also an easy way to make some extra cash that doesn't take much effort on your part.

Copycat recipes are a great way of saving time when you're short on time. They can also help to save money because you don't have to buy ingredients in bulk. Copycat recipes are a great way to save time and money. When you get sick of the same old recipes, just make your own! It's not as hard as it sounds. Copycat recipes are great as long as you follow the recipe exactly. That way, you will get a perfect result every time.

Copycat recipes are a great way to save time and money, they are also a good way to learn how to make a recipe. Copycat recipes are awesome because they allow you to create your own personal food experience. You can try new ingredients and experiment with different flavors, and share your results with the world on social media.

If you're going to make a copycat recipe, don't take shortcuts. It's important to follow the recipe exactly and not change the process in any way.

When you're trying to come up with a copycat recipe, you have to think about the original recipe and how it works. You have to pay attention to the flavors used, ingredients used, and ratios. Nazarian has a book called "Copycat Recipes" that offers copycat recipes for over 60 of his favorite dishes from famous restaurants, and it's available on Amazon. Here are the recipes that we've found:

My advice to you is to try some of the recipes in this post. I have tried many of them, and in my opinion they really work well.

There are many copycat recipe sites out there, but not all of them are created equally. Since the book was published, I've seen a lot of copycat recipes for the book. You can find them on Pinterest, Twitter, and see them in more niche blogs as well. Here are some examples: The most important thing when creating a recipe is to make it taste delicious! Your goal should be to make your recipes so good that you don't even need to make a public recipe.

When your recipe is a big hit, don't feel pressured to share it. If you've been asked for a copy and you're not sure how to do so, ask your followers on social media. You may have noticed that I have a copycat recipe on the blog. This post is my best guess at how to make those recipes so you can save time and money.

Copycat recipes are the absolute best! These recipes give you a taste of a brand, without having to pay the full price. They are usually very cheap and can be made in large quantities.

CPSIA information can be obtained
at www.ICGtesting.com
Printed in the USA
BVHW052107090421
604613BV00005B/124

# Copycat
# Recipes

ISBN 978-1-80183-057-
5269

9 781801 830577